The Deliver Method

The How To Guide on Moving From A Difficult Birth Experience to Manifesting Your Perfect VBAC Story

Willisa Pinney Clarke

Doctor of Pharmacy

To Rubina and Lauris and all the amazing women who have blazed the trail ahead of me. You have taught me well.

- I love you.

Table of Contents

<u>Introduction</u>

Just nursed my newborn baby for the first time today. Our day usually starts around 3 am. Then it's every 2 to 3 hours from there. I look at this beauty and think, I gave birth to her. I manifested this being by visualizing my desires and working towards making them a reality. How did we get here? How did I give birth to this perfect person? (Perfect in my eyes, at least.) She is exactly what I asked for.

This journey started a little over a year ago. I was disgruntled at the medical system after giving birth to my son. Why did I have a c-section on the evening of Halloween 2018? I did the work. Or at least I thought I did. The bills, the care, the fact that my desires were not acknowledged. I felt like I was forced into something I didn't want to do--taken advantage of.

I remember sitting in my hospital bed 48 hours after being told "I couldn't leave." At the time I was 37 weeks pregnant with a healthy, active pregnancy. I followed all the doctor's instructions. I even hired a doula. I sat there reading my doula recommended hypnobirthing book as we waited for something to happen. Progress. Anything that would signal my first child was on the way. I remember skipping to the section on interventions. The section described my current state, exactly. Then it read, "If you've made it to this point, you've gone too far." My heart plummeted. *So you're telling me I could've stopped this? Why were we here? How did we get this far without knowing?* I was tired and heartbroken. I wanted to give birth vaginally, but my body wouldn't open up to let my baby out naturally. We weren't ready. The cascade of interventions were not productive. My mucus plug came out, my water had broken, but we were only at 2cm dilated. For the sake of my baby's health, I agreed to sign papers for major surgery. My cesarean section was a success, and I met my beautiful baby boy. I was a first-time mom basking in the joy of holding my precious baby in my arms for the first time. But I felt unsettled.

I thought back to a week prior. My OBGYN broke the news to me that she had a medical conference planned the week of my due date. She may not be present to deliver my baby. I was hurt. We spent the last 10 months getting to know each other. I asked, greatly disappointed, "Who's going to deliver my baby if you're gone?" Would things have gone differently had she been present?

The months passed, we recovered, normal life resumed, but the unsettled feeling--the regrets--lingered. Did I really need a c-section? Why would the book say "I've gone too far?" A year later I visited the office for my yearly checkup where I intended to bring up my birthing experience. Per usual, my usual OBGYN was out of the office , so I brought it up to her alternate. I couldn't let it go. We had that tough conversation--professional to professional. The look on her face, her inability to respond let me know that my concerns were valid. Something wasn't right about how things went while giving birth. And at that point I decided that the next time would be different. I take responsibility for not fully educating myself as a first-time mom. If I could turn back the hands of time, things would be the same.

I started digging. Researching. I came across the movie titled "The Business of Being Born." I needed to understand what went wrong so I could make it right the next time. I took responsibility for my own actions and circumstances. Honestly, birth is a gift. It's a right. It's my power as a woman. Our power as women. Why are we made to believe we can't do this on our own? The medical system's technology and advancements do have their place. They are designed for emergencies, and they do in fact save lives. But I've found that birth interventions are over recommended and used to please a doctor's schedules and not mom's natural laboring pattern. The business side of "moving things along" causes more harm than good for some.

I wanted to honor my body. I needed to honor my strength. So I started journaling. I needed to get clear on my heart's own needs and desires. What does birth look like for me? Who do I want to give birth to? I got clear on my desires. Then I manifested it. I took action to bring my desires to life...literally!

Birth trauma is oh too common. I wanted change. I needed it to be different. Too many women are taught to believe that once they have a cesarean section, a vaginal delivery is no longer available. Sis, I'm here to tell you **that is not true**. You can make it right for yourself. Holding my second child, a beautiful baby girl, in my arms is proof that it is possible for you. In this book, I outline my three step methodology to manifesting an all natural, empowered vaginal home birth vaginal birth after cesarean (VBAC) approved.

Step 1: Create

As I mentioned, I've broken this magic down into 3 steps. In our first step we explore the world of creation. We were given the power as women to create/bring life. We are the source. Our goal in this section is to manifest what it is that we want. Did you know you have the power to get EXACTLY what you want? Broken into 2 chapters, I'll be teaching you how in these steps.

Chapter 1 will cover the power of deciding. In this chapter, I walk you through journaling, visualizations, and the power of manifestation. We dive in with some journaling prompts and end with the big event. SEX! I navigate all the details to get the job done right the first time. I encourage you to invest in a birth journal. Find a cute composition notebook to write out your thoughts and desires. You can find an inexpensive one at your local big box store.

In Chapter 2 I walk you through how to find the perfect team to support this big, new vision.

Let's dive in!

Chapter 1: Decide

Let's begin by getting clear on what you want. I'm so glad I took time throughout this journey to journal as I recommend you do as well. I'm surprised at what I could make possible once I had faith. Please don't skip this step. This is the most important part. You do not want to miss this. I highly recommend getting a journal to get you started.

Natural birth is beautiful. If you're reading this, more than likely natural birth is something you're considering or curious about. The first thing you have to decide is what is your definition of natural birth? What does natural birth mean to you?

Some examples of natural birth are:

1. A hospital birth without medication
2. A hospital birth with pain medication
3. A birth experience other than c-section
4. A birth in a birthing center
5. An assisted home birth
6. An unassisted home birth

Visualization #1: Imagining what your perfect birth would look like.

Grab a pen and piece of paper. I want you to hone in for a minute. Close your eyes and take a few deep breaths. I want you to write out all your ideas no matter how silly you think they are. Time yourself for 15 minutes and write out anything that comes to mind.

When you're complete, I want you to hold that there, and acknowledge it. When you're done, put it in a safe place. We will come back to it soon.

The importance of envisioning what you want is because soon you'll start reading and hearing stories from other people. I don't want you to get discouraged or out of tune with your own personal desires by listening to everyone else's story. We will do that soon.

Journaling prompt #1: Answer the following question before going to bed.

- What do I want my birth to look like?

Sit on it overnight and come back to the table tomorrow. I highly recommend journaling to keep track of your deepest desires. You can always add to or take away from it later.

Tomorrow we will continue building more on your perfect story. Remember don't rush along. Review your writing upon rising and add any thoughts that may come up as you rest.

Congratulations on completing the most important step. Your experience is going to be magical. Why? Because it's just that. Your Own Desired Experience!

Now it's time to explore the possibilities. This section will help to enhance your experience. I want you to get familiar with the world of birth by looking at other birth stories. I challenge you to look online for positive birth stories. Read through a pregnancy magazine. Watch some positive birth stories on YouTube. Read a few birth blogs on Pinterest. Search ideas: Hospital birth, home birth, natural birth, birth center births, water births, c-section births, cesarean, Pitocin, epidural, unassisted births, doula, VBAC natural birth, midwife birth, and reviews.

Delivering vaginally (anything but a c-section) was always my greatest natural birth desire. Whatever it took to push my child through my vagina and have my husband catch my baby was my biggest dream.

Cascade of Interventions

We are the only species of mammal that doubt our ability to give birth. It's profitable to scare women about birth. Many maternity care interventions are recommended to induce labor or help move things along. Every intervention has unintended effects and are often resolved with further intervention. The cascade of interventions, once initiated, can't be stopped, however. Only 75% of women induced, successfully result in a vaginal birth. That leaves the other 25% with a cesarean birth. They often quickly lead moms away from their dreams and desires for a natural birth. The key to avoiding a sense of defeat is knowing your options and staying true to your deepest desires.

Here's a list of maternity intervention practices:

- Use of various medications to induce labor.
- Artificially breaking the membranes surrounding the baby to release amniotic fluid to initiate or augment labor
- Use of synthetic oxytocin medicine ("Pitocin")
- Use of medications for pain relief.
- Laboring in bed versus being upright and moving about.

These practices disrupt the normal physiology of pregnancy, labor and birth. The truth of the matter is that "the cascade of interventions" is usually just that. One intervention is initiated, which then leads to another and another, oftentimes ending with a c-section. Twenty-five percent of women whose labor was initiated via induction fail to progress and result in a c-section.

The easiest way to birth naturally is to avoid these interventions and allow your body to work its miracle on its own. I need you to get clear on your desires. In chapter

5, we will get into what each intervention entails. We will also explore your options and what to consider should your practitioner recommend any one. Before that, let's work on clarifying a few things. Let's pause for a moment and acknowledge You Are Stronger Than You Know!

Visualization #2:

For this next thought process and visualization, I want you to evaluate your current situation and envision your greatest desire for your next birth experience. For my VBAC mommas, what is it that you want to overcome? What would you like to change from your previous birth(s)? What do you want to be different moving forward?

Based on the interventions listed above, what do you consider going too far? What is a deal breaker for you? Which intervention listed above would be on reserve for absolute emergency only? Which intervention(s) was used on you before? Which would you want to avoid? Which is on reserve if absolutely necessary?

Our ultimate goal with this experience is healthy mommy, healthy baby. We must be mindful that risks may arise. But many times, recommended interventions aren't given in emergency situations and can be delayed. Every birth involves some type of risk, but the more you allow your body to work naturally, the more you lean towards successfully delivering vaginally.

For this visualization I need you to look past all the "what ifs" and hone in right now to your deepest desires in a perfect world.

Journal prompt #2: Despite my fears, what does my perfect birth story look like? What concerns do I have to overcome to make that happen? How will my life change with my new addition?

For this journaling exercise, I would like you to put on some thought-provoking music, set up your timer for about 15 minutes and write out all your thoughts. Acknowledge any concerns. Write it all down. Get clear on your greatest desires and your deepest fears. Again, remember, you are stronger than you know. Honor your strength. Honor your power. Honor your gift and ability to bring life. You were created for this!

Orgasmic Manifestation

Now that we've acknowledged our thoughts and desires, we can now dive into the fun part. Co-creation. Orgasmic manifestation is an intentional manifestation technique to help you create more life-force energy towards the thing that you want to happen. I truly believe that this is what tied everything together for my process, so I highly suggest you give it a go. Seriously, do not skip this!

Step 1: Write out a clear vision for manifestation.

Build upon your birth story desires. Let's explore. Who would you like your baby to be? Boy? Girl? Tall? Short? Look like mommy or daddy? The goal of this step is to establish a clear vision of what you are wanting to manifest or become a reality. Make sure to spend about 10 minutes before you dive into this practice refreshing your mind on what you've written so far. I suggest writing it down or looking at pictures that depict your desires. Feel free to take your time getting clear on your desires before moving forward. The goal of this step is to have a vision for your birth and baby written out in front of you to review before you begin.

Step 2: Work with your partner.

You may do this work with or without a partner. But this is your partner's baby too. Co-creation is a form of collaborative innovation. Ideas are shared and perfected together, rather than kept to oneself. Doing this with a partner will allow more energy to be directed towards your dreams and desires. The more both of you are in agreement on this, the more successful your chances are.

Step 3: Sex.

The main event. I want you to be intentional about this moment. Our ability to conceive happens when we focus on building a heightened state of sexual energy. If getting enhanced (eg. alcohol) is part of your free self, I ask you not to hold back. Loosen up and get comfortable. Work with your magic. Make it fun! What's your favorite way to enjoy foreplay?

Foreplay is a set of emotionally and physically intimate acts between two people meant to create sexual arousal and desire for sexual activity. It can include kissing, sharing fantasies, or touching one another's genitals. Foreplay adds to your sexual excitement and helps prepare a woman's body for intercourse, which increases vaginal lubrication.

You may consider your ovulation date. Ovulation is required for implantation. But I want you to focus more on building your sexual energy. The goal of this step is to achieve a good orgasm. A good orgasm allows sperm to move up and through the cervix easily. I've found tracking ovulation to add stress to the dynamic.The more time and effort spent charging up your sexual needs enhances the enjoyment of lovemaking and successful implantation. Enjoy this time!

Step 4: After ejaculation, tilt your hips upwards using several pillows.

Step 5: Trust the process. Embrace your partner. Lay there for a while and embrace the moment. Hug yourself, honor your body, know that your desires are on their way.

Chapter 2: Your Perfect Team Blueprint

We continue Step 1: Create.

In this chapter, we cover the importance of having a VBAC and natural birth supportive team. You've worked so hard to get to this point. I want you to celebrate. Have you planted the seed to the manifestation of your vision yet? Regardless if you've confirmed pregnancy or reviewing the book to prepare for your next pregnancy, I want you to feel proud for taking steps so far to honor yourself and your desires.

Now we need to find the perfect team to support your vision. Having the proper support team is immense and can make or break your chances of having a VBAC and successful natural birth. You have some big decisions to make in this chapter. I want you to approach them with knowledge and peace.

Before we begin I would like you to take some time to watch the documentary film entitled "The Business of Being Born." This film breaks down the birthing system and the cause and effect of our maternity care interventions. You'll be surprised how much more empowered you will feel after watching this. Understanding this will regrant more than half of your God-given birthing power.

When it comes to delivering a baby, there are 4 provider options to choose from. Let's begin with a few definitions, shall we?

1. **OBGYN** (Obstetrics and gynaecology) is the medical specialty that encompasses the two subspecialties of obstetrics and gynecology. Obstetrics deals with all aspects of pregnancy, from prenatal care to postnatal care. An obstetrician can also provide therapies to help you get pregnant, such as fertility treatments. Gynecology is the medical practice dealing with the health of the female reproductive system. The term means "the science of women." Gynecologists give reproductive and sexual health services that include pelvic exams, Pap tests, cancer screenings, and testing and treatment for vaginal infections. They diagnose and treat reproductive system disorders such as endometriosis, infertility, ovarian cysts, and pelvic pain. Obstetrics is the surgical field that deals with childbirth and includes cesareans, whereas gynecology is the field of medicine concerned with women's health, especially their reproductive health. OBGYN's have a large umbrella of women to care for.

2. **Family medicine** is a medical specialty devoted to comprehensive health care for people of all ages.

The specialist is called a family physician or family doctor. They are pretty old school but can provide care for the entire family. Some deliver babies and go on to caring for the newborn, the mom, and all members of the family.

3. A **licensed professional midwife** is a trained health professional who cares for mothers and newborns around childbirth, a specialization known as midwifery. The education and training for a midwife is similar to that of a nurse. A midwife helps healthy women during labor, delivery, and after the birth of their babies. Midwives may deliver babies at birthing centers or at home, but most can also deliver babies at a hospital. Midwives only care for the pregnant woman. Midwives usually take a holistic and woman-focused approach to pregnancy and childbirth; many work with the backup support of a medical doctor.

4. A **certified nurse-midwife**, or **CNM**, is an advanced care registered nurse who gives care and counseling during pre-conception, pregnancy, birth and postpartum. CNMs also provide primary health care centered on women and their families all through their reproductive lives.

After my first OBGYN cesarean delivery, I decided to work with a certified midwife for my second pregnancy. Here's why:

Reason 1: OBGYN's have a large umbrella of women to care for and are trained surgeons. Most want to have control over the way they practice and therefore oftentimes recommend emergent and not so emergent interventions. After my first interview with my midwife, she explained to me that the most effective way to a successful VBAC is to not be touched (receive no interventions). It is very important to evaluate if your chosen provider is against VBACs, VBAC supportive, or VBAC tolerant. OBGYN's that are pro natural birth are usually prideful about their success. It's important to evaluate where your provider stands because you don't want to be sabotaged into going against your truest desires. This is why I began the book with your very important birth visualizations. I highly suggest you ask questions at consultation visits early in pregnancy to evaluate each provider's likelihood of intervening in a woman's natural labor pattern. I've included a few questions for visits below.

Reason 2: Florida law bans women who have had cesarean births from birthing in a birth center. Therefore if I wanted to be "untouched," I would have to attempt giving birth naturally at home. I suggest you get familiar with the laws in your area and consult your provider. Note: You may have to travel a bit outside of your area's jurisdiction. But for me, a second cesarean was a non-negotiable, unless absolutely medically necessary, so I had decisions to make. I had to decide: 1) to give birth au naturale at home with a patient, knowledgeable midwife or 2) find a VBAC supportive OBGYN. Honestly, I felt if I allowed my body to work on its own without the added temptation of having options available, I could be successful at giving birth vaginally. So I mustered up the courage and decided to be all in for my all natural at home water birth. My advice to you: know yourself, evaluate your deepest desires, needs, and weaknesses, compare and contrast the providers available in your area and then choose wisely. Consider what you want to change from your last birthing experience. What left you feeling disconnected? First time moms, you don't know how your body labors yet, but consider what would produce a happy birthing experience for you, uniquely.

If you are low risk and leaning toward a water birth or hypnobirthing, an experienced midwife is who I'd suggest looking into. But regardless of risk, if you'd be more comfortable with a medical doctor providing your care, or desire high-tech equipment readily available, then an OB-GYN or family doctor might be the best fit. I highly advise you to interview a few providers in your area to assess how they interact with you, their expertise and comfort level with VBAC and/or natural birth and their willingness to make you feel listened to.

<u>A few other side notes</u>

During your interviews by phone or in person, consciously be aware of providers whose medical stance do not align with your ultimate desires. You are worthy of being fully supported on this journey, so honor your intuition and feel free to look around for other available providers. Also, if you are currently under the care of an OBGYN, who has provided your care for some time and you feel comfortable with their service, I highly encourage you to still ask the questions included below. You want to learn how they practice and ascertain their perspective on supporting women through a VBAC and birthing naturally. You want to ensure that your chosen provider is aligned with all your desires and needs.

Interview questions for providers as a candidate for labor support:

1.) How many of your patients have had medication free births? (Don't use the word natural because some providers think natural and vaginal mean the same thing)

2.) What is your c-section rate? (If they don't know these statistics, they're not good.)

Red flags

Be aware of feeling guilted into hiring a certain provider. A lot of times we unconsciously choose an OBGYN because it's the route that most women take. They have access to high-end equipment. Also they are medical professionals. However, I want you to take some time to reflect on your options and how you intuitively feel before making a decision.

Why I Loved My Midwifery Experience

I truly enjoyed and highly prefer the midwife model of care. The birthing center provides a more laid back setting where the atmosphere felt more cozy with less white coat syndrome. My midwife visits were usually about an hour long at her homebase birth center and a few home visits were included as well. I loved that my midwife made time to check on my overall wellbeing. She had a guide of questions that we reviewed at each visit, which allowed her to do a thorough review of my emotional, physical, and mental health between visits. This was in addition to the procedural listening to the baby's heart rate, tracking your weight, and testing urine samples. I found it much easier to answer questions versus trying to write down and remember questions in between visits.

On each of my visits I felt seen, heard, and understood. The visits felt like all care and attention was focused on my desires and needs. In my OBGYN experience, it was a bit different. I had less time with the doctor and didn't always have an opportunity to ask all of my questions.

As a career-focused mom, having someone take the time to ask questions, thoroughly evaluate me, and listen to me made all the difference! I left every visit feeling strengthened with a game plan for caring for myself and my growing baby.

Doula - Mothering The Mother

A doula is the most important support person that you can have for your big day. Doulas are professionally trained birth coaches who "mother the expectant mother". There are several types of doulas that provide different levels of care, but at this time we will focus on the benefit of having a birth doula. A birth doula offers prenatal education and emotional support, and she advocates for the mother. She is not a medical professional, but she is well trained and well primed in the protocol for childbirth whether at home, in the hospital, or at a birth center. She is a liaison between the medical practitioners and the expectant mother. After losing my mom at the age of 25, birth support was something I seriously desired. Having a good doula was profound in helping me to feel super supported beyond what my spouse (or your support partner) could provide on the big day.

Doulas are worth their weight in gold. A doula's sole focus is to support you and your needs. While your birth practitioner focuses on keeping the baby safe and sound, your doula will support you through the majority of labor. Your doula helps you prepare for and cope with labor pains. They usually meet with and start laboring support with mom at home. They provide suggestions and support for moving and breathing through contractions. Some may also provide services by phone.

You might be thinking, "I've got my partner at my side; he'll care for me." Keep in mind that the birth experience can be extremely emotional and surreal for him, too. He might not be well equipped to handle the level of emotional care that you need on your big day. (I talk about how to get your partner prepared for the big day later on, so keep reading.) The doula provides reassurance to the partner and helps facilitate communication between the mother and her partner. Doulas can also tag team with the partner to provide labor support to the mom so that the partner gets to rest when he needs to. This is important! Your partner needs rest as well. A doula understands the importance of the birth experience, so she aims to help make sure those memories are as positive as possible.

Doulas are also helpful in reducing medical risks. Women who have doulas present at birth tend to have shorter labors with fewer complications and less of a need for caesareans, Pitocin (a drug which induces labor), and other medical interventions, such as pain medication or an epidural.

Warning! Not All Doulas are Created Equal.

I met my perfect doula after my first birth, as I considered using her services for placenta encapsulation. Due to several reasons, I decided not to ingest it but bury and plant on top of it instead. She showed up to my doorstep with cookies and my placenta and we connected instantly. She was super compassionate, she was a woman of color (as am I), and her energy was so genuine and radiant. She also had tons of clients who she guided through a natural home birth. She really held space for me as I was still quite emotional about how my last birth experience went. I explained that my water was low during my first pregnancy, which led to a long spiral of undesirable interventions. She took the time to listen; then she apologized. She apologized on the doctor's behalf and affirmed that it didn't have to go the way they did, and working together things, would be different in my next pregnancy. Her apology felt genuine and reassuring, even encouraging me to not let what happend break me because I though I could not alter the past, I could impact the future. This was powerful. I didn't know this lady at all, but she planted the seed of natural birth deep down in my heart. I kept her number close, and she was one of the first people I contacted when I found out I was pregnant with my second.

I must say though, not all doulas are created equal. As with your birth practitioner, I highly advise you to interview and choose a doula wisely. The experience with the doula I used for my first birth wasn't so favorable.

Don't be afraid to invest in yourself. Trust your gut! Then choose the right fit for you. I will go more into detail about my VBAC doula's assistance in chapter 5: The Experience. But in the meantime, let's do some more exploring, shall we?

Visualization #3: Spend some time rereading and reflecting back to your visualization #2. Now I want you to envision how you are supported? Who do you envision around you? Are you moving around freely at home, or are you in a room at the birthing center or maybe a hospital room with all the beeps and fancy machines? What is it that you need to feel supported? Are your support people breathing with you, massaging you, feeding you ice, juice, water, snacks? Are you dancing, singing, meditating, praying, doing yoga, stretching, walking? Are you allowed to eat? What are you wearing? Do you have a birth pool? What about a shower?

Journal prompt #3: Which provider best fits your needs? What are you looking for in a doula? What type of labor support will you need? Who's personality and experience am I most confident with? VBAC experience? Natural birth tolerant or supportive?

Remember, you are the decision maker and you are allowed to get what you want.

<u>Chiropractic Care</u>

Chiropractic care is considered safe and effective during pregnancy. Routine chiropractic care helps manage pain in your back, hips, and joints. It also helps with establishing pelvic balance which provides your baby with as much space as possible over the course of your pregnancy. As a pharmacist, I stand on my feet for 12 - 13 hours on a work day. I found visits to my Webster-certified chiropractor throughout my third trimester of pregnancy very beneficial. Balancing the pelvis is important for the baby to be able to descend through the birth canal.

Of course you know I'm going to challenge you to find a provider that fits. When looking for providers in your area, ask a friend or try google searching "webster-certified chiropractor near me". In conversation, try learning more about their experience of working with women desiring an all natural birth. Have they had a natural birth before or maybe their wife or close friend or family member? It'll be more beneficial if your provider has experience with natural birth or VBACs. Knowledge is power and having someone to support you in this way is super beneficial. I also found it beneficial for my chiropractor to have a flexible schedule. Coming down to the last days, it was easy for me to call in for a same day appointment.

The chiropractor I was referred to was absolutely phenomenal. She had given birth naturally in the comfort of her home 4 times. That's correct. FOUR! And she was not afraid to share stories and motivate me by saying "You are stronger than you know." My chiropractor was super beneficial to my natural birth success. I looked forward to her appointments because not only did she adjust me, but she gave me a pep talk every time. She poured life into me at every visit by sharing inspiration, rooting me on, and pumping me up to stay strong and trust the process. I wish I could share my Jackie with everyone, but in lieu, I sprinkle some Jackie dust on the page to let you know that
YOU CAN DO IT!
Now go out there and find you a Jackie!

Supportive Partner

Your supportive partner is another very important member to your support team. Your support partner can be your spouse, a family member or friend. This person is super important because more than likely they are with you throughout pregnancy and will be with you on the big day.

And guess what momma? We need them to be ready! Ready to support you and ready to give you what you need. More than likely, they got you here in the first place, right? So let's get them strong, prepared, and ready for the big day as well.

A knowledgeable support partner opens doors for a more empowering experience. Because your support partner is with you throughout pregnancy, here is a list of ways they can support you before the big day:

- Help with meal planning and ensure fruit and vegetable intake daily
- Stock up on water
- Take you out for walks (if weather permits)
- Check in and follow up after prenatal visits
- Fetch those infamous cravings
- Massage your back, feet, hips and legs
- Allow space for intentional alone time
- Set up furniture pieces and help prepare the nursery
- Help to stock up on postnatal household needs
- Care for older children
- Budget for expenses

<u>Preparing Your Support Partner For The Big Day</u>

As I mentioned, your support partner is a significant part of your birth team. You want them to be prepared too. Their most important job is to keep momma relaxed. Dimmed lights, soothing music, smiles and affirmations are welcome. Have water, drinks and snacks readily available. Your support partner may guide you through some progressive muscle relaxation exercises or even a relaxation exercise. They can gently massage your head or back and hold your hand during those really rough contractions. I suggest they read up on the stages of labor. I've found that the most beneficial way to get your partner involved is to educate them with some birth education. I recommend a natural birth course in Chapter 3 for those dads who want to be all in.

The "Mama Natural" natural birth course is so highly recommended that it has its own section in chapter 3. The course is very thorough and has support partner training integrated within each section. You may find this to be a fun training for both of you to do together as your belly grows. The course also includes moves that you and your support partner can do together. Check them out by typing the following URL exactly as it appears in a browser on your phone or computer.

mn.ontraport.com/t?orid=667894&opid=1

But if your spouse/support partner is anything like mine, whatever I'm signing him up for has to be an hour or less. Most partners just want to be told what to do and where they can help. So sit with that thought for a minute and journal in the next journaling prompt on how you would like to be supported. Then relay that message to your support partner. Add to that list as needed anytime something comes up.Then allow them to show up while acknowledging their emotions as well. Cheers to happy, healthy families!

Visualization #4: I want you to visualize yourself on the big day. Imagine yourself in your chosen location with your chosen practitioner. If you chose to hire a doula, how would you like them to team up with your support partner? How is your support partner supporting you? Are they singing to you? Swaying with you? Breathing with you? Where are your other children? Hiring or requesting care? How are you working together throughout pregnancy? Mentally make a list of things you want to accomplish before the baby arrives.

Journal Prompt #4: What type of support will you need from your support partner? What do they need to know or be able to do to best support you? Write out that list of things to accomplish before the baby arrives. Let them know how to touch, breathe with and talk to you.

Now that we've secured our support team, we shift our focus to step 2: Embrace. Let's jump over to Do The Work.

<u>Step 2: Embrace</u>

By this time we have established our pregnancy and are now changing our focus to doing all the things necessary for maintaining this healthy and happy pregnancy experience. We will dive in a bit more by adding one more special person to your support team. Then we will review the health and nutrition tricks I followed to take me through to the finish line. We then finish off with birth education to get you knowledgeable about birth. All of step 2 will be covered in chapter 3. Let's dive in!

Chapter 3: Do The Work

Hire A Wellness Coach

I had the pleasure of hiring a holistic nutritionist and gut health expert prior to my pregnancy. More support, you may ask? Well, let me explain.

So far we've worked through all the support we need for our birth. We got our midwife or OB to check on the baby, we've got our doula to prepare for and coach us through labor pains, we've got the chiropractor keeping our hips and pelvis aligned, and we've got hubby or our support partner working on keeping our system working while preparing for this dynamic change. But what about health beyond motherhood? What about our own wellbeing? Our mental and emotional wellbeing? This is why you need a wellness coach.

My coach was super supportive in helping me to work through many of my own issues. She helped prepare me physically and mentally for our new addition and life change. She taught me how to integrate clean and unprocessed nutrition into my day to nurture myself and ultimately my baby. She served as an accountability partner, while holding big space for me to expand and discover myself and my needs. Creating space for my baby was one major task we worked through together as well. Having her allowed me to decide what I wanted and work towards it. She even held me accountable to write you this book.

My coach was paramount in helping me to feel as if business shall proceed as usual while adding a baby to the mix. As a career-focused momma, this was super important to me. If this resonates with you, momma, I get it. And I'm here to support you. Making babies is one of our superpowers, but I've got so much more to give, so much more for you to receive. So if making babies isn't your only superpower, I encourage you to hire a coach that will keep you grounded and accountable in the other areas of your life.

Looking back, I think of all the things my coach and I worked through. Women are pregnant for an average of 40 weeks (10 months). And if you remain committed, you can use this time to really take charge of some things.

As a NLP practitioner my coach helped me heal old subconscious wounds by doing inner work, such as inner-child healing. We focused on breaking down barriers and obstacles that were causing me to hold myself back. She was profound in holding me accountable to things I promised myself to work through. As a career-focused mom, I often get distracted or discouraged when I feel overwhelmed. Having someone by my side, cheering me on, and holding my hand was instrumental in ensuring that I took care of myself too.

Balancing work, home, hubby, and the kids often leaves moms feeling as if they are drowning under all the obligations. Hiring a coach can help. I initially hired my coach to help me lose weight. But having a balanced and organized life was what I really needed. The healing helped me to discover that, then we were able to get to work on other areas. In the 10 months of pregnancy leading up to the big day I was able to do the following:

- I worked on healing my relationship with food and using it to honor my body. Therefore I simply focused on filling myself up on what was good instead of sorting through what was bad.
- I worked on healing my relationship with exercise. I simply began to focus on movement instead of the all or nothing 30 minutes in the gym everyday. This allowed me to integrate enjoyable things such as dance or neighborhood family walks throughout the week.
- I worked on *remembering* myself at work. It was so easy to focus on getting the work done that I sometimes would delay eating, drinking water or using the bathroom.
- I honored myself by understanding that I can't pour from an empty cup. I created time for me to reflect, meditate and honor my thoughts daily.
- I made time to reorganize my walk-in closet and create a working system for bills, documents and the mail. We created a working schedule around my

busy schedule to find pockets of time for the things that were holding me back. I was gracefully able to check off a few important tasks in my life.

I did all that while creating life, caring for my son, managing a pharmacy, working my side hustle, and making time for God and hubby. I share all this to inspire you and grant you the permission to ask for additional help.

If any of this sounds like support you would need, I highly recommend a wellness coach to assist with tangible emotional support throughout your pregnancy journey. You may find more information on my coach by visiting her website at caprisharichards.com.

Nutrition and Wellness

Nutrition

Consuming healthy nutrition is super important during pregnancy. Despite cravings and/or appetite changes, I've narrowed down a few simple steps to help you during pregnancy:

The 80/20 rule is a great guide for your everyday diet. Here, you focus on consuming nutritious foods 80 percent of the time and enjoy a serving of your favorite treat with the other 20 percent. It's like eating healthy and having your cake too!

For the 80%, I challenge you to focus on filling up on plant-based whole foods such as whole grains, veggies and fruits. Throughout pregnancy, I focused on having a small salad daily with lunch and consuming one serving of fruit as a snack daily. These simple measures were trackable, achievable, and easy to integrate into my busy lifestyle. It allowed me to cover the bases by ingesting digestible nutrients that were good for me and baby.

What beats the cravings? Having what you desire! Throughout pregnancy I craved french toast & pancakes, Cold Stone's Founder's Favorite, brownies and tons of sweets. It was very important to create structure around my 80% so indulging in my 20% didn't feel so guilty.

<u>Hydration</u>

Hydration is super important during pregnancy and one factor very near and dear to my heart. Not drinking enough is probably one of the most detrimental things you can do to your body and your baby. Your amniotic sac contains amniotic fluid which sustains your baby during gestation. Your body's muscular system requires it for maximum function. Your heart, pelvic floor and legs have muscles that need hydration. Water also helps with balancing the vaginal flora and preventing yeast infections. It stimulates the kidneys to flush out toxins.

Please hydrate! Even if it means sacrificing efficiency at work or otherwise to stop for bathroom breaks. I committed to drinking 1.5 liters of water daily by finding a 1.5 L bottle on the shelf at my local grocery store and committed to finishing the bottle daily before going to bed. You can do the same. Whatever you decide, keep it simple sweetie!

<u>Movement</u>

Elevating your heart rate through exercise is important for training your body to move oxygen and blood to your baby and your body's organs faster. As a career-focused working mom, I oftentimes beat myself up to stay committed to a workout program or gym schedule. With my second pregnancy, I decided to simplify my perspective on exercise by focusing on simply moving every day. This helped to cut out the pressure of committing to a specific thing and opened doors for exploration. I discovered enjoyable ways to move that include family neighborhood walks, intentionally dancing to my favorite songs, taking dance classes, watching prenatal yoga on youtube, and participating in an online prenatal barre class. The main idea is to commit to doing something everyday. Movement is important for keeping mommy's body healthy and keeping baby happy, healthy, and in position.

<u>Coping with Morning sickness</u>

Pregnancy comes with its share of discomforts with morning sickness and nausea being one of them. Morning sickness affects 70-80% of pregnant women and can greatly impact your ability to perform certain activities. Here are a few tips to help you through.

- Sniff a fresh scent to override scented triggers
- Hydrate
- Focus on small meals and snacks
- Catch a breath of fresh air by taking a slight stroll
- Stretch your arms above your head and breathe

- Suck on ginger mints or sip on ginger tea
- Speak to your provider about medications that can help

Morning Routine

I found it super beneficial to integrate a morning routine that allowed me to create intentional time for myself daily. This session took about 15 minutes and helped to keep me grounded and gratitude focused.

I started with a devotional of some sort for spiritual guidance. I then put on some soft music and set my timer for 5 minutes. I used my birth journal daily and headed each page with the date and 'gratitude list'. In the first 5 minutes I wrote out everything that came to mind that I was currently grateful for on that day. I followed that by heading the next section with 'Future Gratitude List' and wrote everything that came to mind that I was already thankful for having, even though technically I didn't have them yet.

Looking back, you'll be surprised at how important an attitude of gratitude is for repositioning your mind on something, especially now as you prepare for your perfect birth.

Journal Prompts #5

I encourage you to do a 5-minute gratitude list daily. Here are a few other topics to journal on throughout pregnancy. The topics below help to acknowledge where you're at and evaluate where you'd like to be.

Week 8: Moms, what would you like to be different in this pregnancy? Both moms and first time moms, based on information presented so far, how can you make this the best pregnancy journey ever?

Week 10: Moms, what do I have to heal from to make this pregnancy right?

Week 12: Would I like to know the gender of my baby? And why?

Week 20: Halfway there! Celebrate!! Am I doing all I can for the betterment of myself and my baby? What can I improve?

Week: 30: Single-digit-countdown time. What else do I need to feel ready?

Week 40: If you've made it this far, congratulations! You are almost there!! What do I need most to allow myself to relax, surrender and release?

<u>Sample What I Eat In A Day</u>

Breakfast:
2 boiled bananas
Jamaican ackee cooked down with peppers and onions
Boiled egg
Half an avocado
Lemon water
Celery juice

Mid morning snack:
apple, watermelon, tangerine, or handful of mixed nuts

Lunch:
Small garden salad (lettuce, spinach, olives, carrots, tomato, mushroom, cucumbers, red onion)
Homemade lasagna: Ground turkey, mixed veggies, whole wheat pasta, mushroom spaghetti sauce, cheese

Afternoon Snack:
Tangerine, banana, or a piece of dark chocolate

Dinner:
Basmati rice
Red kidney beans
Baked chicken wings
Mixed vegetables

<u>*Natural Birth Class*</u>

One of the requirements to work with my midwife was to enroll in a natural birth class. Although childbirth education was included in my doula's package, I found the virtual course referred to below as super beneficial. This birth course is a bestselling online childbirth class, brought to you by the #1 natural parenting brand, and has added so much value and contributed to building my confidence for my birthing success. The content, the affirmation cards, the beautiful beaded bracelet handmade in Haiti, the professional advice of a midwife throughout, Genevieve's expertise in giving birth naturally 3 times, and seeing numerous natural birth videos made all the difference in building my confidence for doing birth naturally. This birth course was so beneficial that I've partnered with them to get a special price just for you. Type the URL below exactly as it appears in a web browser on your phone or computer and check them out today.

mn.ontraport.com/t?orid=667894&opid=1

I want you to take your time through each class and learn all you can to confidently birth naturally. Have your support person join in as well as Genevieve was awesome at integrating advice for them throughout the course.

If interested in signing up for their free pregnancy week-to-week email series, use the URL included below.

https://wk2wk.securechkout.net/?orid=667894&opid=14

Visualization #6: Imagine a world where you have overcome all the things holding you back. What things have you let go? What is now established and set in place as a result?

Journal Prompt #6: What are some things you would like to work through before your life changes again? Evaluate your current status of self care? Food? Movement? Head space? Do you need to outsource emotional support? What's needed for you to feel your optimal self?

Step 3 - Deliver

So we've made it to the final step: Deliver! Momma, it is almost time to meet your baby and I bet you can't wait! In this step, I teach you what to do in the last few months of pregnancy to allow yourself to flow, expand, and let your baby out into this world. In chapter 4 we speak about preparing for the big day. I break down how to prepare your home, rest and get your mind right. I suggest having all these things ready and in place by week 36. In chapter 5 I review my experience and provide you a guide to get all you desire on the big day. Understanding the stages of labor (explained in a natural birth course) will help you to recognize the changes in your body as you progress through the stages of labor. Let's dive in.

Chapter 4 - Preparing For The Big Day

How To Prepare Your Home

For this birth, I really wanted to be ready. With the COVID pandemic supply shortage and my first pregnancy ending at 38 weeks, I started preparing for the big day around month 6. I suggest you start gathering things from the list below around month 6 or 7 with a goal of having them all on hand by week 36. This checklist may not be thorough but it covers a pretty good bulk of needs. It can be used as a guide to ease your mind and be prepared for the first 4 weeks after having baby. When purchasing items on the list be mindful of your usage to ensure you pick up enough for now and 2-4 weeks beyond. I also suggest you try taking time off from work before baby arrives to finalize any last minute duties.

Home Supplies (* indicates item specific for home birth)

- rolls of paper towel & toilet paper

- fresh towels (used to replace old towels that may get dirty during birth)*

- plastic shower curtains to protect bedding (purchase an extra one if you have carpet)*

- an extra set of bed sheets*

- hydrogen peroxide

- alcohol

- toiletries: deodorant, soap, toothpaste, toothbrush, lotion

- pads: 1 pack of overnight and 1 pack of what you regularly use

- laundry supplies (laundry detergent, softener, dryer sheets, etc)

- stock up on fluids (water, coconut water, gatorade, alkaline water)

- stock up on snacks (fruits, tangerines, grapes, blueberries, bananas, pineapple, granola bars, yogurt, mixed nuts, trail mix, z-bars)

- easy breakfast ideas (eggs, oatmeal, dry cereal)

- stock up on easy prep meal items (beans, rice, pasta, freezer meals, frozen veggies)

- meal prep and freeze a few meals

<u>Plan a Baby Shower</u>

Hosting a baby shower is a creative way to share the news and allows family and friends to pitch in and ease the out-of-pocket expenses for the expecting parents.

- Create a registry (eg. Amazon, Target, Walmart, Buy Buy Baby)
- Add items you will need (diapers, car seat, clothes, crib, bassinet, swing, stroller, toys, etc.)
- Decide if you would like to do it virtually or in person
- Pick a date, choose a theme and create an invite (use Pinterest for inspiration)
- Find an online host (zoom, google hangout) or location (home, conference center, park)

- Plan decorations, games, and meals if necessary
- Maybe some music
- Start on time and have some fun

<u>Self care</u>

- catch up on wellness checks (dentist)

- what about that hair? (easy styles, supplies needed, braids, locs, hair ties, hair bands)

- Nails & Pedicure

- Waxing

- organizing your space

- check the mail

- put bills on autopilot or pay a month or two ahead (mortgage or rent, light, water, cellphone, cable, pay up birth bills thus far)

<u>Nesting</u>

- Hire cleaners (clean bathrooms, vacuum carpet, rugs, and living room furniture, sweep, mop, change bedding, wipe down countertops)
- Set up furniture and prepare baby's room
- Wash, organize and pack away baby's clothes (newborn and 0-3 months)
- Verify that you are stocked up on baby supplies (baby soap & shampoo, diapers, wipes, onesies, sleep n plays, hats, socks, mittens, baby laundry detergent, baby lotion, baby blankets, baby formula)
- Planning to breastfeed? (nursing bras, nursing pillows, all natural nipple cream, does your

insurance cover a pump?, learn about getting a good latch, and watch how to breastfeed videos)

The more organized and peaceful your space feels, the easier it'll be for you to flow and fall into character. Labor requires a certain state of mind. It's a place of complete surrender. So the more items on your list are checked, the more you can allow yourself to just be. Be persistent and keep at it!

Rest

Resting is very important throughout pregnancy. At times, you may have little energy and your growing belly is taking up more room than usual these days. So I want to ensure that you are resting. Aim to get a good night's sleep (6-8 hours) and/or take naps. Having the proper pillows can help you to rest comfortably. You can look into purchasing a pregnancy pillow or a C-pillow. If you have extra bedroom pillows, place one under your belly and one behind your back for support as you lay on your side. Avoid laying flat on your back.

Allow yourself the opportunity to put your feet up sometimes. Lay and watch tv or listen to music. We are focusing on reducing stress on the body. Remember your body is sustaining two complete individuals with one rapidly changing day by day. In between it all, be sure you make time to catch your breath every once in a while.

Get Your Mind Right

I remember at this time, calming tracks were very helpful. I used YouTube hypnobirthing tracks to fall asleep at night. I did breathing exercises and third trimester prenatal yoga. We also walked a lot. I found the affirmation cards included with the birth course referred to at the end of Chapter 3) to be very helpful. I found that the 15 minute daily morning routine and journal prompts (explained in Chapter 3) helped to keep me grounded and in a happy space. You are so close to the finish line. Trust that your baby will be in your arms soon.

Quick composure exercise

I found the following exercise to be helpful in preparing me mentally for what contractions feel like. I want you to grab a small bag (like a sandwich-sized ziploc) and some ice. Put the ice into the bag. Get a timer (there may be one on your phone) and set it for one minute.

Hold the bag of ice in your hand, start the timer and close your eyes until the timer goes off. It's just one minute.

Whew. That was tough. One minute seems like it'll never end. But you made it. Celebrate.

I want you to do that again. But before you begin, put on music that you like. Something beaty, flowy, soft and melodic.

Now, close your eyes and visualize yourself on a beach watching the water calmly go in and out. If the beach scene isn't relaxing for you, visualize yourself somewhere that feels calm.

Hold the bag of ice in your hand, start the timer, and close your eyes again. Listen to the music, visualize yourself on that beach and hold it there until the timer goes off.

Now how was that?

Did the time go faster when you were on the beach listening to music?

How a contraction feels

A contraction can feel like you're holding ice. They also last for just one minute or less. A contraction can also be described as waves in the ocean. The pain intensifies but then dissipates. Some are really intense and others not so much. Your body's combination of oxytocin, melatonin and endorphins make contractions almost euphoric. A contraction can't be stronger than you because it is you.

Birth affirmation: I can do anything for one minute.

My goal for this section is to prepare you mentally for relaxing, zoning out, surrendering and disengaging your body. The more you allow your body to work with your contractions, the faster you allow your body to release your baby. Practice makes perfect. The easier it is for you to get to that state on game day, the quicker you get to meet your baby.

So while you're waiting for labor pains to begin, I want you to constantly reflect back to your perfect birth story. The one we created in step one. Feel the feels, get in the zone, get into character, set up the scene, lay out your clothes, do all the things. Be ready.

Then TRUST! Your baby will be in your arms soon.

Journal Prompt #7: What do you expect a contraction or surge to feel like? How do you plan to cope? Are you still fearful of birth? What support do you need to overcome that fear?

Chapter 5: The Experience

We are here! Let's dig in. As I write this book, I reflect back to my own Perfect Birth Story journal prompts and realize I was blessed to get an experience exactly as I manifested or desired things to go. It was sometime between May 11th and May 15th. We still hadn't found out the sex, but I was confident it was a girl. Ask and it shall be given unto you, right? Both hubby and I wanted a princess to complete our palace.

The Waiting Game - Prodromal Labor

I start this chapter with this topic because it is highly undiscussed. It is also the stage of labor that drove me the craziest. Based on conversation, I realized that this is also the stage where most women go into the hospital, start being monitored, and are offered to start that famous cascade of interventions explained in Chapter 2. In my birth story, I requested that in this second pregnancy I experienced how it felt to go all the way. I actually made it to 41 weeks and 4 days before meeting my baby girl.

Many apps and pregnancy resources talk about Braxton Hicks. Braxton Hicks are known as false labor pains or practice contractions because the womb is actually practicing by contracting and relaxing. Not all women will have Braxton Hicks contractions. And if you do, you'll usually feel them during the second or third trimester. Braxton Hicks are completely normal. My labor may have started with Braxton Hicks at 41 weeks, but things progressively intensified over the next few days.

Prodromal labor started for me at 41 weeks. I made it to 40+ weeks of pregnancy calmly and without pain. At this point, my midwife and I agreed to initiate natural labor inducing techniques because laws in Florida don't allow her to monitor me beyond 42 weeks. The first thing we tried was acupuncture. Labor prep acupuncture and acupressure is one of the best kept secrets of Chinese medicine. Acupuncture kicked my body into gear and I started having subtle labor pains in my lower back two days later. My body was in labor for 5 days. Yes, 5 days! But as explained above, it progressively got worse. I will discuss my labor experience more in a bit, but first let's dive into prodromal labor.

Prodromal labor is labor that starts and stops before fully active labor begins. It's usually caused by something called 'cervical effacement', thinning, or ripening. It's often called "false labor" but this is a poor description. Medical professionals recognize that the contractions are real, but they come and go and labor may not progress. Prodromal labor often starts and stops at the same time each day or at regular intervals, and many moms will call their birth team or go to the hospital thinking it is real labor. In some cases it can last several days or weeks before active labor begins.

Labor can be different for each woman. At the start of labor, most women report cramping, period type pains and lower backache which slowly progresses into bouts of irregular contractions lasting a few hours. <u>This is normal.</u>

In layman terms, I would describe prodromal labor as turning a key in your car's ignition but the car not turning over to start. The goal is to turn the key until the car starts, then shift the car into gear, and drive away. You want labor to start, intensify, and push your baby out. But with prodromal labor, your body doesn't fully kick into gear. Don't be mistaken though, something is happening, but some women's bodies, like mine, process this phase slowly.

Oxytocin, the body's labor intensifying hormone is augmented at night due to the body's melatonin. This causes most women to go into labor at night. In the late evening, your body surges with melatonin (the sleep hormone). This fabulous hormone interacts with oxytocin to promote contractions. Because melatonin is the hormone that is responsible for encouraging us to go to sleep, it clearly reaches its peak during the dark hours, making us more likely to start contracting in the evening.

Prodromal labor was a major part of labor for me. My body would intensify at night but calm down in the day. Could you imagine how it felt to go to sleep with contractions day after day at 40+ weeks thinking this might be it. Then wake up the next day thinking, "Dang, I'm still pregnant." Honestly, I almost wanted to throw in the towel and drive myself to the hospital. The only reason I didn't was because I couldn't figure out a way to get home by myself after major cesarean surgery. (Funny, not funny.) Hubby wasn't with it, my entire team was 100% onboard for a natural birth, COVID numbers kept increasing, and I was stuck. I kept my vision of my perfect birth story at the forefront and pushed through.

Yes mama, I know you are tired. But, trust me, your baby will be in your arms soon.

<u>When To Go To The Hospital or Call The Midwife</u>

411: You start making ways to the hospital when your contractions are 4 minutes apart, lasting for 1 minute long for an entire hour.

<u>How to Survive Prodromal Labor</u>

1. Labor at home as long as tolerable or until above guideline (411)
2. Download a contraction tracker. Track contractions for 30 - 60 minutes at a time.
3. Eat well, stay hydrated, use the restroom often, and keep yourself focused on other things, besides the contractions.
4. If you would normally be working, try to get some work done to keep yourself busy. I suggest working on busy work type projects. You've got a list of assignments in chapter 4. If all of those are completed, you may work on coloring a birth coloring book.
5. If you would normally be sleeping or resting, try to get some sleep or rest as you are going to need it.

It's preferable for you to lay on your left side for optimal blood circulation to the baby. At this point, my midwife allowed me to have one 6 oz glass of wine only after dinner or 2 OTC Benadryls to help me to calm my nerves. (Consult with your provider for guidelines on what they allow.)

6. You can walk slowly around the house or even in your neighborhood to help your labor progress and keep things moving in the right direction.

7. Monitor the baby's activity by doing kick counts.

8. Keep in close contact with your team. Your provider may need to perform cervical checks to monitor your progress.

9. Keep in mind that things may move slowly and take days or move quickly and turn over within hours. Be ready!

10. Repeat steps 1 - 9 until labor progresses, pain is intolerable, you feel rectal pressure, contractions meet the 411 criteria, or if you notice something abnormal.

Stages of Labor

Early labor refers to contractions that are irregular and brief (30 - 45 seconds). Mom is able to talk through contractions. Not much pain relief help is needed. 0 - 4 cm dilated.

Active Labor - contractions are more regular and longer (~ 60 seconds long). Must breathe, vocalize, or focus deeply during contractions. Pain management tools needed. 5 - 8 cm dilated.

Transition - mom is well into active labor. Contractions may feel like they are one on top of the other. Cervix is completely dilated. At 10 cm baby starts to descend and pass the pubic bone. Shortest but most painful part of labor. Toilet sitting very helpful. Sitting in your birthing tub could really help with surges at this time.

Baby Delivery - phase where you can push. Once baby is ready to exit, your body gives you a primal urge to push. Pushing can take some time.

Placenta Delivery - phase after baby is delivered when the placenta exits the vagina

Cascade of Interventions continued

So if a hospital birth is something you've decided on, I highly recommend you get familiar with the following list of terms. Most first time mothers go into the hospital hoping for the best, anxiously awaiting the moment they meet their babies. Most first time moms are also unaware of possible circumstances and uneducated on their options. Here is usually where the medical system infuses fear. Honestly, it's more profitable to scare women about birth.

Once a woman approaches her final stages of pregnancy, doctors begin to throw about certain terms indicating a possible need to hurry things along. I've heard terms such as low fluid, big baby, breech baby, small pelvis, and risk of shoulder distortion; just to name a few. Every type of birth includes some type of risk. But it's key to trust that you will know when it's crisis mode or not.

<u>Quick Breakdown of Medications and Procedures Used in Labor</u>

Anyone planning a hospital should know these terms:
- Labor Inducing Medications and Procedures
    - Cytotec (Misoprostol)
    - Pitocin is the synthetic version of the body's natural hormone Oxytocin that causes the uterus to contract. It is given intravenously in the arm in small amounts to induce labor and ripen the cervix. Unlike Oxytocin, Pitocin does not pass the blood brain barrier therefore once initiated the body's natural endorphins aren't properly activated to provide a natural response of pain relief.
    - Cervidil (Dinoprostone) is the only FDA-approved vaginal insert for cervical ripening. It's inserted high in the vagina next to the cervix to mimic your body's natural prostaglandins. Prostaglandins help your cervix gradually soften, thin, and dilate naturally.
    - Foley bulb
- Breaking of the membranes
- Pitocin (synthetic Oxytocin) can also be used in combination with labor inducing medications to

strengthen labor contractions during childbirth or to control bleeding after childbirth. Pitocin can cause your contractions to start off stronger and faster than they would if labor began naturally. That has the potential to put added stress on your baby as well as your uterus.

- Medications for pain relief
    - Systemic Analgesics
        - Opioids
        - Nitrous oxide (Laughing Gas)
    - Anesthesia
        - Local anesthesia
        - Regional anesthesia
            - Epidural - most common type of pain relief used for childbirth in the United States. The medication is given continuously through a tube placed in the lower back and injected into the epidural space around the spinal cord. It creates a band of numbness from the bellybutton to your upper legs but you remain awake and alert. Most common side effect is generalized itching. Requires a urinary catheter and limits movement once inserted.
            - Spinal block

- Combined spinal-epidural (CSE) block
- General anesthesia
- Laboring in bed versus being upright and moving about

If you've decided to go with a hospital birth, it's important for you to understand the terms explained above. Reflect back to your birth story created in visualization and Journal Prompt #1. If labor has begun, allow yourself time and space to reground and remind yourself of your birth desires. You've bought this book, you've invested time and effort. A+, Momma! You are educated, you have the power, you've got this. If you've done the work, you and baby are safe, and you feel properly supported. Allow yourself to breathe through every love (Oxytocin) hormone surge. Work with your body. BREATHE! You will meet your baby soon!

As I mentioned, every type of birth includes some type of risk. There are risks and side effects associated with all the medications and procedures listed above. But what I don't like about the options above is some medical staff force themselves onto moms and start to recommend them before they are necessary. Many times completely not needed if moms are given time to labor. This causes some moms, despite giving birth to healthy babies, to walk away from their birth experience feeling disappointed in themselves and their bodies.

The disappointment can be coined "birth trauma" and it's the most common but unspoken aftereffect of a medically intervened birth. Birth trauma is a shorthand phrase for post-traumatic stress disorder (PTSD) after childbirth. While trauma can be physical, this trauma is often emotional and psychological. Birth trauma includes what happened during labor and birth and how mom is left feeling afterwards.

Momma, the labor pains you feel or are about to feel are real. But they are also temporary. And you get a beautiful reward at the end of it! Embrace that. Then believe in yourself and know that you can do it. You've been given the powerful ability!

There are several different ways to help your body move things along naturally. In the next section I'll explain.

Natural Ways To Induce Labor

Red Raspberry Leaf (RRL) Tea

Red Raspberry Leaf (RRL) Tea contains the alkaloid fragrine which helps to strengthen the uterus and pelvic area. I started drinking Red Raspberry leaf tea in my third trimester. But, with the approval of your practitioner, you may start drinking a cup a day as early as the second trimester.

Dates

Dates are thought to increase cervical ripening, reduce the need for a medical labor induction or augmentation, and reduce postpartum blood loss. I started consuming 6 dates daily around week 36. I loved blending them in a smoothie with almond milk, peanut butter, and banana. I enjoyed this as a snack regularly.

Pineapples

The popular theory is that somehow the bromelain from the pineapple makes its way to your cervix and causes the breakdown of tissue there. This in turn causes the cervix to soften and stimulate labor. I bought a whole pineapple, cut it into chunks, and ate it as a snack in week 40.

Evening Primrose Oil

Starting at 38 weeks, I placed an Evening Primrose Oil softgel deep into my vagina at night to work directly on the cervix while I slept. Evening primrose oil is thought to help the cervix soften and efface. Some studies suggest that the linolenic acid triggers a prostaglandin response that can help shorten labor duration. I used EPO up until 4 days before delivery when I lost my mucus plug. You can use EPOas long as your water isn't broken and there is no vaginal bleeding.

Acupuncture

Acupuncture has been used in Chinese Medicine for thousands of years and should be administered only by a licensed acupuncturist. It is believed to balance the *chi* or vital energy within the body. It might also stimulate changes in hormones or in the nervous system. Acupuncture at 41 weeks helped to get my labor started.

Nipple Stimulation

By the morning of day 2 of prodromal labor, my contractions had spaced out to about 30 minutes apart. At this point my midwife had ordered me to do a few rounds of nipple stimulation with a breast pump. Please consult your practitioner before attempting to do this.

Nipple stimulation mimics breast-feeding and causes sensory cells in the nipples to signal the brain to release oxytocin. Some women use a breast pump to stimulate the nipples. Others may prefer to use their hands or a partner's mouth for stimulation. Stimulating the breasts may help bring on full labor by making contractions stronger and longer. Rubbing or rolling your nipples helps the body release oxytocin. As previously mentioned, Oxytocin plays a role in arousal, initiating labor, and bonding between mother and child. This hormone also makes the uterus contract after labor, helping it return to its pre-pregnancy size.

Acupressure

Acupressure is another Chinese medicine technique that's based on the concept of life energy which flows through "meridians" in the body. I agreed to signing up for a labor inducing acupressure massage on day 3 of prodromal labor. By applying pressure to specific points amongst the body, blood flow to my uterus increased, hormonal responses were influenced, and uterine contractions were stimulated.

Miles Circuit

The acupressure masseuse performed a technique on me called spinning babies. This series of positions makes birth easier by improving fetal positioning which reduces the chance of cesarean. Your practitioner or doula may be able to help. Check out spinningbabies.com for more information.

Stripping of the membranes

Things really started to pick up for me after my labor inducing acupressure massage. So much so that although my contractions were still pretty spaced out, they were definitely intensifying. On Christmas Eve (day 4 of labor), my midwife came by for a visit and performed a cervix check. I made it to 3 cm. We agreed to strip the membranes, a procedure also known as a membrane sweep. It involves your practitioner sweeping their (gloved) finger between the thin membranes of the amniotic sac in your uterus to induce labor or move things along. The procedure is a little uncomfortable but breathing through it and having a compassionate provider could help.

Bounce on an Exercise Ball

I spent most of Christmas Day in what felt to be early labor. Hubby, big boy and I enjoyed the time indoors by watching tv, bouncing on the exercise ball, playing toddler games, eating a hearty dinner with a glass of wine. Gently bouncing on an exercise ball to induce labor encourages the baby to move down making contact with the cervix to dilate.

Tips on how to use the exercise ball: 1) Sit on the exercise ball, with your legs wide apart, move your hips up and down; then sway from side to side. 2) With your support partner sitting behind you on a couch or bench, lean back between their legs and allow them to help hold you in place as you sway your hips left and right on the ball. You can also do circles. Try these moves for 20 minutes, changing directions periodically. 3) Alternate abdominal lifts (lifting up your belly) with circles on the ball between and during contractions.

<u>Sex</u>

Babies, technically, come out the same way they go in and sex can induce labor in several ways. Sexual activity, especially after having an orgasm, can release oxytocin, which may help to jumpstart uterine contractions. For pregnant people who have sex with men, there are prostaglandin hormones in semen that help ripen the cervix. Third time's a charm! Three sessions are equal to 1 Cervidil.

The prostaglandins in hubby's sperm helped to kick my body into active labor. Unbeknownst to me, I spent the night of Christmas in active labor. I had spent so many nights tracking contractions and in pain that at this point that I had a higher pain tolerance.. (In the next section we speak about pain coping techniques.)

The morning after sex, the day after Christmas, my midwife called to check in. I was miserable. I hadn't slept all night. I had no appetite. I made it to the morning again, my contractions spaced out, and my labor stalled. She requested I go to the chiropractor for a visit, then come in to get checked. She checked me and I was at a whooping 7 cm with a bulging bag of water. I did it! I was officially in active labor. Whew, all that pain counted for something.

So now standing at the birthing center, 7 cm dilated, this baby could be delivered any minute now. My midwife ordered me to hurry back home, and my team met me there.

<u>Movement and Exercise</u>

Reflecting back to my perfect birth story vision written in May 2020, I manifested walking as a way I wanted to pass the time during labor. The family and I took daily neighborhood walks once maternity leave began. I integrated curb walking by walking to the edge of the sidewalk and lifting myself into a high knee with each step. Up until hours before delivering my baby, while stalled at 7 cm dilated, my team and I walked the neighborhood to catch some fresh air before the sun set and we got back to work.

When women give birth in the movies, they are generally portrayed one way: lying down, in bed. Research shows that moving freely in labor improves a woman's sense of control, decreases her need for pain medication, and may reduce the length of her labor. Exercise can be anything that gets the heart rate up. And even if this method doesn't work, it's a great way to relieve stress and keep your body strong for the task ahead.

There may be other ways to induce labor not mentioned above, but I told you what I used. This list is a great place to start. Feel free to search online for others or consult with your practitioner. And keep in mind, every step is a step in the right direction. Breathe! Trust! Your baby will be in your arms soon.

Tips for Helping a Laboring Woman

Darkness and Soft Lighting

Bright light can suppress the brain's production of melatonin. Suppressed production causes lower melatonin levels in the bloodstream subsequently decreasing oxytocin. Keep it nice and low. Fill your space with lamps or candles.

After coming back from our walk, we created a space of calm serenity. Darkness with low lighting helped to create that space for me.

Music

Music really helped me cope with labor pains. I found soft melodic, relaxation music very beneficial. It helped me to zone out and get some rest at night. I listened to hypnobirthing tracks and yoga music. Upbeat music was fun for dancing and car rides. Someone recommended I listen to this group of girls with beautiful voices called Beautiful Chorus. Listening to them was super beneficial in coping through early and active labor. (Check them out on Spotify or Youtube.)

<u>BREATHE</u>

How to breathe through a contraction (on your own):

1. Pay attention to how surges feel when they start to come on
2. Have your timer easily accessible to hit when the feeling begins
3. Begin breathing deeply. Inhale, then exhale.
4. Don't hold your breath.
5. Keep breathing deeply.
6. You can do anything for one minute!

How to breathe through a contraction (partner assisted):

1. Mom pay attention to how surges feel when they start to come on
2. Have your timer easily accessible to turn on when you feeling starts to begins
3. Support partner find a position where you can look mom into the eye. This can be standing, bending, or sitting in front of her.
4. Hold her hand or face to get her attention through touch. This helps her feel your presence.
5. Demonstrate a slow, controlled breathing rate.
6. Stay with her through it until it is over.

7. Affirm her! Say things like, "You're doing great," "You're so strong", "I'm proud of you", "One wave at a time", "On to the next one".

8. Support her. Have her sip water, get a snack or lay and get some rest.

<u>REST</u>

I know you're excited! I know you want to try hurrying things along. But don't do it. The best thing you can do for your body in the early stages of labor is rest. Once you get to active labor you won't be able to rest, and you will need all of your strength then. Ignore surges for as long as you can. Lay and watch movies in the daytime and rest at night. Time contractions for about 20 - 30 minutes at a time then turn it off and get some rest.

<u>Water</u>

Drinking water, sitting in water, standing in water (shower) are all helpful for coping with labor pains. I found water therapy to be my thing! Taking a shower in the morning after a long night helped to get me up and ready for the day. Laying in the tub with candles and soft music was great for allowing time to pass.

<u>The Big Day</u>

Then the birth pool. My birth pool was literally my perfectly designed removable epidural. Once we returned from our walk, my doula set up my birthing pool. We labored for a bit until things really picked up. My doula held my hand and/or looked me in the eye and helped coach me through every contraction. Just as I explained how to breathe in the section above. I put on my swimsuit top and got in the pool. Everyone around, anxiously awaiting, then surges completely stopped. I found the birth pool to be super relaxing. Sitting in water was very good to me. It created room for me to breathe.

I got out and we started working again. My midwife checked me, I was at 8 cm and stalled again. We tried the miles circuit again. My doula and midwife worked together to come up with a plan to help me progress. They guided me through the miles circuit and used different techniques to help jumpstart my labor again. With patience and time the feeling came upon me to get up, move around, find a safe space and hunker down. I made it to the shower, then the pool. It had been a few hours, the water in the pool had cooled down too much for the baby, she was coming quickly, so I had to get out and lay on the bed. I felt the urge to push. With all my might, working along with my body, I gave it my all. Push 1. I felt her hair. I waited for that urge again. Push 2, her head popped out. The entire room drew silent in awe. I heard hubby giggle and whisper, "Oh my, it's her head." We waited again for the next surge and Push 3, right into hubby's hands she popped out into this world! She was out! Straight into hubby's hand just as I manifested it. I did it! We did it! I couldn't believe we finally made it to the end. This beautiful prize was all worth it!

The moment had finally arrived. Peace, tranquility, darkness, calm, quiet was all needed right then. Support at its best. I allowed myself to fully receive and be fully supported. I surrendered. I allowed myself to be. In my strongest power. My God-given goddess energy was finally activated.

Visualization #8: Create a vision of your perfect birth. Combine all the elements from each visualization. Add in your induction and coping techniques. Research and be confident in your decisions.

Journal prompt #8: Write it all out!

If birth has happened already: Congrats! Journal on how it turned out! Did you get all your desires? What would you have done differently?

Final Notes

Thank you for joining me on this journey. Thank you for sticking it through to the end. I'm hopeful that you trust the process and receive the dreams of your life as well. One thing I must mention though is that my c-section scar didn't affect me one bit. The possibility of uterine rupture practitioners scare you about is very rare, occurring in less than 1% of women who attempt a vaginal delivery after cesarean. This should put your mind at ease that the odds are definitely in your favor!

There are so many things I've overcome since manifesting my perfect birth story. I realized that this technique can be applied to many areas in life. Manifesting my daughter's birth motivated me to allow myself room to dream, hope, believe more is possible than I once imagined. To go beyond limitations. Now I place no limits on what I can accomplish. This journey is a launching pad to visualizing more desires and feeling empowered to flesh them out. I want the same for you. I want to inspire a generation of strong women. Women who have always existed, who I simply help open the proverbial curtains, revealing the strength they already possess within. Strength from our creator. Be encouraged that you have within you what it takes to experience the birth and life you've always longed for. As the saying goes, "If you can conceive it, you can achieve it!" That goes for your desired birth journey...and so much more!

About the Author

Willisa Pinney Clarke is a Black Caribbean woman, wife, mother of two, pharmacist and author. Originally from the Virgin Islands, Willisa has built a career in pharmacy and currently practices as a doctor of pharmacy in Florida. After having her first child, Willisa questioned the integrity of the medical system when her birth resulted in a c-section. Amidst the COVID pandemic, Willisa manifested a way to change things about her first birth and created a way to feel more in control of her birthing experience. The journey resulted in her successfully giving birth to her beautiful baby girl au naturale in the comfort of her home.

Based on her own experience, Willisa shares the inside scoop about her birth experience and provides her ultimate step-by-step method to manifesting your perfect baby and birthing experience.

This guide is for all the mommas who yearn to take control over their birthing experience, and desire to give birth naturally regardless if they've had a c-section before (VBAC) or not.